The Super Easy Bread Baker Cooking Guide

Simple And Tasty Sweet & Savory Bread Maker Recipes For Beginners

Jude Lamb

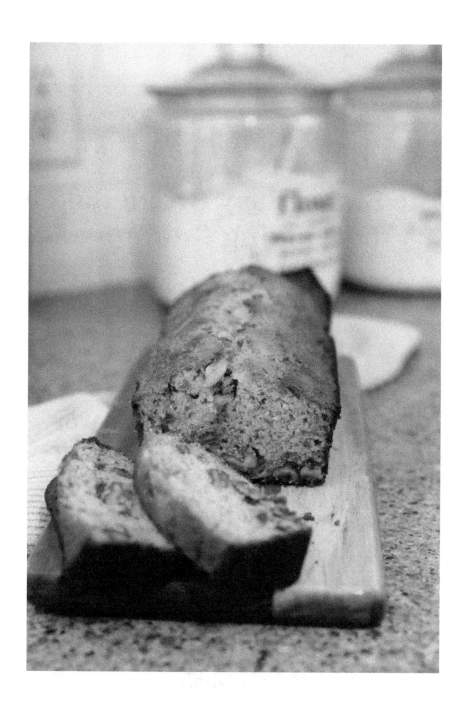

Table of contents

Making Bread

There is nothing like the scent of freshly baked bread to greet you when you wake up. Bakers traditionally produced their products during the early hours meaning their loaves were fresh, hot, and mouth-watering tasty for hungry customers wanting a slice of bread to go with a slap-up breakfast.

Bread historically dates back to Neolithic or even prehistoric times in its earliest incarnation.

Prime ingredients include flour and water used to make the dough. The dough can have numerous additives to offer assorted consistency, flavors, and healthy preferences. Additives may include yeast, fat, salt, baking soda, fruits, spices, eggs, milk, sugar, or vegetables. You can even add seeds to the bread, oils, and nuts. Bread is quite a versatile product and can be devoured on its own or as an accompaniment to the main dish. The dough is traditionally baked, but modern alternatives could include steaming.

The outer part of the bread, commonly known as the crust, can be baked into a hard or soft version. The inner part of the bread is classed as the "crumb," strangely not the small bits that cover your lap.

The prime time to eat a loaf of bread is soon after it has been removed from the oven. At this delicious time, the bread is warm, aromatic, and fresh. Leaving the bread for any length of time will cause the bread to become stale.

A quirk dating back to the 13th century was the Baker's Dozen.

A Baker's Dozen, ironic as it was from the 13th century, relates to 13 items making a dozen instead of the usual 1 1/2. As history would have us believe, a Baker's dozen suggested that punishment was administered to bakers who short-changed their customers. One way to ensure that a customer always received a full quota was to give more bread than paid for. Furthermore, if one loaf was damaged, burnt or was of unacceptable quality, there were still 1 1/2 loaves available for the customer.

Another explanation of the Baker's Dozen, and slightly more believable, is that when round loaves were placed on a standard baking tray, the configuration was 3+2+3+2+3 which gave a greater density to the tray and allowed easier stacking.

Over the decades, the baking of bread has followed the path of many traditions updated to reflect the changing needs of society. Whereas bread was always the preserve of the local baker, modern supermarkets now have their own "in-house" ovens, and bread is baked to suit customer demand.

Cauliflower Tortillas Bread

Preparation Time: 6 minutes

Cooking time: 21 min

Servings: 5

Ingredients:

- 3/4 big head cauliflower (or two cups riced)
- 2 large eggs (Vegans, sub flax eggs)
- 1/4 cup cleaved crisp cilantro
- 1/2 medium lime, squeezed and zested
- Salt and pepper, to taste

Directions:

1. Preheat the stove to 375 °F., and line a heating sheet with material paper.
2. Trim the cauliflower. Cut it into little, uniform pieces, and pulses in a food processor in groups until you get a couscous-like consistency. The finely riced cauliflower should make around 2 cups pressed.
3. Place the cauliflower in a microwave-safe bowl and microwave for 2 minutes, then mix and microwave again for an additional 2 minutes. In the event that you don't use a microwave, a steamer works similarly. Place the

cauliflower in a fine cheesecloth or slender dishtowel and dry up as much fluid as could be expected, being careful not to burn yourself. Dishwashing gloves are recommended as it is extremely hot.

4. 4.In a medium bowl, whisk the eggs. Add cauliflower, cilantro, lime, salt, and pepper. Blend until all combined. With your hands, shape 6 little "tortillas" on the material paper.

5. Bake for 10 minutes, cautiously flip every tortilla, and put back to the stove for an extra 5 to 7 minutes, or until totally set. Place tortillas on a wire rack to cool marginally.

6. Heat a medium-sized skillet on medium. Place a prepared tortilla in the container, pushing down somewhat, until dark-colored —for 1 to 2 minutes on each side. Do the same way with the remaining tortillas.

Nutrition:

- Calories: 30
- Carbohydrates: 8 g
- Net Carbohydrates: 2.5 g
- Fiber: 7.5 g
- Fat: 8 g
- Protein: 10 g

Herb Focaccia Bread

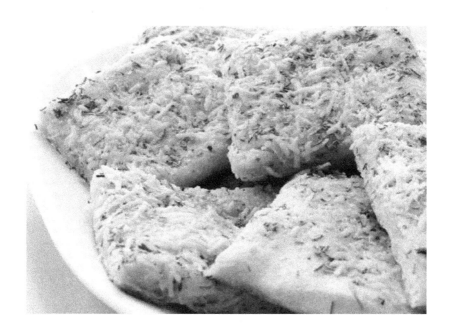

Preparation Time: 3.5 hours

Cooking time: 45 minutes

Servings: 8

Difficulty: Expert

Ingredients:

Dough:

- 1 cup water
- 2 tablespoons canola oil
- 1 teaspoon salt
- 1 teaspoon dried basil

- 3 cups bread flour
- 2 teaspoons bread machine yeast

Topping:

- 1 tablespoon canola oil
- ½ cup fresh basil
- 2 garlic cloves (to taste)
- 2 tablespoons grated Parmesan cheese
- 1 pinch salt
- 1 tablespoon cornmeal (optional)

Directions:

1. Put all the bread ingredients in your bread machine, in the way they are listed above —starting with the water and finishing with the yeast. Make a well in the middle of the flour and place the yeast in the well. Make sure the well doesn't touch any liquid. Set the bread machine to the Dough function.

2. Check on the dough after about 5 minutes and make sure that it's a soft ball. Add water —1 tablespoon at a time if it's too dry, and add flour— 1 tablespoon at a time if it's too wet.

3. When the dough is ready, put it on a lightly floured hard surface. Cover the dough and let it rest for 10 minutes.

4. While the dough is resting, chop the garlic and basil, grease a 13x9 inch pan, and evenly sprinkle with cornmeal on top of it.
5. Once the dough has rested, press it into the greased pan. Drizzle oil on the dough and evenly sprinkle with the salt Parmesan, garlic, and basil.

Nutrition:

- Calories: 108
- Carbohydrates: 37.4 g
- Fiber: 1.6 g
- Fat: 7.3 g

- Protein: 7.7 g

Sugar-Free Cream Cheese Frosting Bread

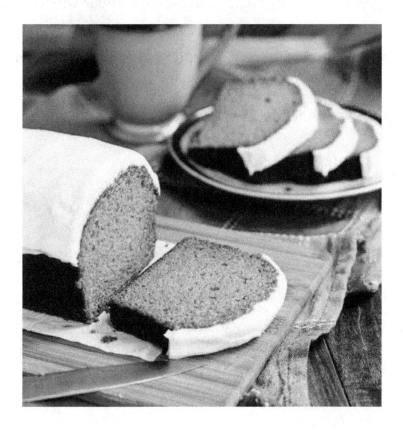

Preparation Time: 5 minutes

Cooking time: 10 minutes

Servings: 6

Ingredients:

- 4oz cream cheese

- 2 tablespoons butter, cubed, softened

- 1/2 cup erythritol, powder, or granulated

- 1 teaspoon vanilla extract

- 1 tablespoon heavy cream

Directions:

1. In a mixing bowl, combine cream cheese, butter, vanilla, and erythritol. Mix using a hand mixer.

2. Add in heavy cream —1 tablespoon at a time until it reaches a smooth consistency.

Nutrition:

- Calories: 12

- Carbohydrates: 9 g

- Protein: 2 g

- Fat: 11 g

Cheese and Bacon Bread Loaf

Preparation Time: 1 hour

Cooking time: 45 to 50 minutes

Servings: 10

Ingredients:

- 1/3 cup sour cream
- 4 tablespoons melted butter
- 1 ½ cups almond flour
- 1 cup grated cheese
- 1 tablespoon baking powder
- 2 large eggs
- 7 ounces bacon

Directions:

1. Preheat oven to 300°F. Line the loaf pan with baking paper.
2. Cut and dice the bacon and cook until crispy.
3. In a bowl, mix almond flour and baking powder with a fork.
4. Using a hand mixer, cream the sour cream and eggs into the flour mix. Add to the mixed dry ingredients along with cooled butter and combine well.
5. Add the grated cheese and cooked bacon into the dough.

6. Empty the dough into the bread loaf pan. Sprinkle the top with extra cheese if you want the bread to be extra cheesy.

7. Bake in the oven for 45 to 50 minutes.

8. Cool, slice, and serve.

Nutrition:

- Calories: 292
- Fat: 13 g
- Carbohydrates: 4 g
- Protein: 3 g

American Cheese Beer Bread

Preparation Time: 5 minutes

Cooking time: 60 minutes

Servings: 8

Ingredients:

- 1 ½ cups of fine almond flour
- 3 teaspoons of unsalted melted butter
- Salt, one teaspoon
- 1 egg
- 2 teaspoons swerve sweetener
- 1 cup Keto low-carb beer
- ¾ teaspoon of baking powder
- ½ cup of cheddar cheese, shredded
- ½ teaspoon of active dry yeast

Directions:

1. Prepare a mixing container, where you will combine the almond flour, swerve sweetener, salt, shredded Cheddar cheese, and baking powder.
2. Prepare another mixing container, where you will combine the unsalted melted butter, egg, and low-carb Keto beer.

3. As per the instructions on the manual of your machine, pour the ingredients into the bread pan, taking care to follow how to mix in the yeast.

4. Place the bread pan in the machine, and select the Basic bread setting, together with the bread size and crust type, if available, then press Start once you have closed the lid of the machine.

5. When the bread is ready, using oven mitts, remove the bread pan from the machine. Use a stainless spatula to extract the bread from the pan and turn the pan upside down on a metallic rack where the bread will cool off before slicing it.

Nutrition:

- Calories: 80
- Fat: 1.5 g
- Carbohydrates: 13 g
- Protein: 3 g

Jalapeno Cornbread Mini Loaves

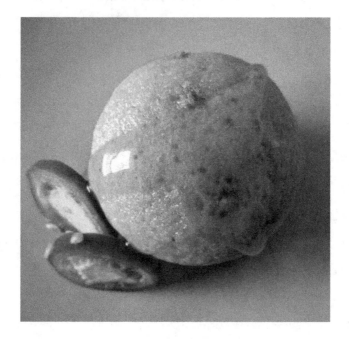

Preparation Time: 16 minutes

Cooking time: 21 min

Servings: 5

Ingredients

<u>Dry Ingredients:</u>

- 1 ½ cup almond flour
- ½ cup brilliant flaxseed feast
- 2 teaspoons heating powder
- 1 teaspoon salt

<u>Wet Ingredients:</u>

- ½ cup full-fat harsh cream
- 4 tablespoons softened spread
- 4 large eggs
- 10 drops fluid stevia
- 1 teaspoon Amoretti sweet corn separate
- ½ cup ground sharp Cheddar
- 2 new jalapenos, seeded and films removed*

Directions:

1. Preheat the stove to 375°F. Set up a smaller than expected portion dish (8 portions) by spraying with cooking oil or greasing with margarine to avoid sticking.
2. In a large bowl, whisk together the dry ingredients including the almond flour, brilliant flaxseed feast, preparing powder, and salt.
3. In a medium bowl, whisk together the wet ingredients. Blend the wet and dry ingredients together, and then add the diced pepper and ground cheddar into the hitter.
4. Spoon the hitter equally into the readied portion pan. Top each portion with a pepper ring to garnish.
5. Bake for 20-22 minutes or until the portions begin to turn brilliant and darker.
6. Cool the portions in the search for gold for 5 minutes and afterward transfer to a wire rack to wrap up.

Nutrition:

- Calories: 230
- Carbs: 4 g
- Net Carbohydrates: 1.5 g
- Fiber: 9.5 g
- Fat: 10 g
- Protein: 5 g
- Sugars: 3 g

Italian Blue Cheese Bread

Preparation Time: 3 hours

Cooking time: 30 minutes

Servings: 8

Ingredients:

- 1 teaspoon dry yeast
- 2 ½ cups almond flour
- 1 ½ teaspoon salt
- 1 tablespoon sugar
- 1 tablespoon olive oil
- ½ cup blue cheese
- 1 cup water

Directions:

Mix all the ingredients. Start baking.

Nutrition:

- Carbohydrates: 5 g
- Fats: 4.6 g
- Protein: 6 g
- Calories: 194

Bacon Jalapeño Cheesy Bread

Preparation Time: 5 minutes
Cooking time: 40 Minutes
Servings: 12

Ingredients:

- 1 cup golden flaxseed, ground
- 3/4 cup coconut flour
- 2 teaspoons baking powder
- 1/4 teaspoon black pepper
- 1 tablespoon erythritol
- 1/3 cup pickled jalapeno
- 8 oz. cream cheese, full fat
- 4 eggs
- 3 cups sharp cheddar cheese, shredded + 1/4 cup extra for the topping
- 3 tablespoons Parmesan cheese, grated
- 1 1/4 cups almond milk
- 5 bacon slices (cooked and crumbled)
- 1/4 cup rendered bacon grease (from frying the bacon)

Directions:

1. Cook the bacon in a large frying pan, set it aside to cool on paper towels. Save 1/4 cup of bacon fat for the recipe, allow to cool slightly before using.
2. Add wet ingredients to the bread machine pan, including the cooled bacon grease.
3. Add in the remaining ingredients.
4. Set the bread machine to the Quick bread setting.
5. When the bread is done, remove the bread machine pan from the bread machine.
6. Let cool slightly before transferring to a cooling rack.
7. Once on a cooling rack, top with the remaining Cheddar cheese
8. You can store your bread for up to 7 days.

Nutrition:

- Calories: 235
- Carbohydrates: 5 g
- Protein: 11 g
- Fat: 17 g

Almond Flour Bread for keto diet

Preparation Time: 7 minutes

Cooking time: 15 min

Servings: 7

Ingredients:

- 1 ½ cups almond flour
- 6 large eggs separated
- 1/4 cup butter, softened
- 3 teaspoons heating powder
- ¼ teaspoon cream of tartar it's alright on the off chance that you don't have this
- 1 squeeze pink himalayan salt
- 6 drops liquid stevia discretionary

Directions:

1. Preheat broiler to 37
2. Separate the egg whites from the yolks. Add Cream of Tartar to the whites and beat until delicate pinnacles set.
3. In a food processor, mix the egg yolks, 1/3 of the beaten egg whites, melted margarine, almond flour, preparing powder, and salt (Adding ~6 drops of fluid stevia to the mix can help lessen the mellow egg taste). Blend until

combined. This will be an uneven thick batter until the whites are added.

4. Add the remaining 2/3 of the egg whites and pulse softly until well mixed. Be careful not to over mix as this is the mixture that gives the bread its volume!

5. Pour blend into a buttered 8x4 portion dish. Cook for 30 minutes. With a toothpick, check if the bread is cooked through.

Nutrition:

- Calories: 210
- Carbohydrates: 9 g
- Net Carbohydrates: 2.5 g
- Fiber: 5 g
- Fat: 10 g
- Protein: 9 g

Bacon Breakfast Bagels Bread

Preparation Time: 7 minutes

Cooking time: 15 min

Servings: 8

Ingredients:

- ¾ cup (68 g) almond flour
- 1 teaspoon thickener
- 1 large egg
- 1 ½ cups ground Mozzarella
- 2 tablespoons cream Cheddar
- 1 tablespoon spread, softened
- Sesame seeds to taste
- 2 tablespoons pesto
- 2 tablespoons cream Cheddar
- 1 cup arugula leaves
- 6 cuts flame-broiled streaky bacon

Directions:

1. Preheat stove to 390°F.
2. In a bowl, combine the almond flour and thickener. Then, add the egg and blend into a single unit until very well combined. Put in a safe spot. It will resemble a raw ball.

3. In a pot, over medium-low warmth, gradually melt the cream cheddar and mozzarella together and remove from heat once softened. This should be possible in the microwave as well.

4. Add your softened cheddar blend to the almond flour blend and mix until all combined. The Mozzarella blend will stick in somewhat of a ball, yet don't stress, endure with it. It will all, in the long run, mix well. It's imperative to get the Xanthan gum fused through the cheddar blend. On the off chance that the mixture gets too extreme to even think about working, place in the microwave for 10-20 seconds to warm and rehash until you have something that looks like batter.

5. Split your mixture into 3 pieces and fold into round logs. On the off chance that you have a doughnut skillet, place your logs into the container. If not, make hovers with each log and consolidate and place it on a preparing plate. Make sure you have decent circles. The other method to do this is to make a ball and level marginally on the heating plate and cut a hover out of the center in the event that you have a little cutout.

6. Melt your margarine and brush over the highest point of your bagels and sprinkle sesame seeds or your desired garnish. The margarine should enable the seeds to stick. Garlic and onion powder or Cheddar causes decent

increments on the off chance that you to have them for flavorful bagels.

7. Place bagels on the stove for around 18 minutes. Watch out for them. The tops ought to go brilliant dark-colored.

8. Take the bagels out of the stove and permit cooling.

9. If you like your bagels toasted, cut them down the middle the long way and spot them back in the stove until somewhat brilliant and toasty.

10. Spread bagel with creamy cheddar, spread in pesto, include a couple of arugula leaves, and top with your fresh bacon (or your filling of decision.)

Nutrition:

- Calories: 90
- Carbohydrates: 4 g
- Net Carbohydrates: 2.5 g
- Fiber: 4.5 g
- Fat: 8 g
- Protein: 8 g

Collagen Keto Bread

Preparation Time: 5 minutes

Cooking time: 15 min

Servings: 8

Ingredients:

- 1/2 cup Unflavored Grass-Fed Collagen Protein
- 6 tablespoons almond flour (see formula notes beneath for without nut substitute)
- 5 fed eggs, isolated
- 1 tablespoon unflavored fluid coconut oil
- 1 teaspoon sans aluminum preparing powder
- 1 teaspoon thickener (see formula notes for substitute)
- Pinch Himalayan pink salt
- Optional: a spot of stevia

Directions:

1. Preheat broiler to 325 ° F.
2. Generously, oil just the base piece of a standard size (1.5 quarts) glass or clay portion dish with coconut oil (or spread or ghee). Or on the other hand, you may use a bit of material paper, cut to fit the base of the dish. Not oiling or

covering the sides of your dish will enable the bread to stick to the sides and remain lifted while it cools.

3. In a big bowl, beat the egg whites until firm pinnacles structure form. Put in a safe spot.

4. In a small bowl, whisk the dry ingredients together and put them in a safe spot. Add the discretionary spot of stevia in case you're not an enthusiast of eggs. It'll help compensate the flavor without adding sweetness to your portion.

5. In a little bowl, whisk together the wet ingredients — egg yolks and fluid coconut oil, and put in a safe spot.

6. Add the dry and the wet ingredients to the egg whites and blend until well combined. Your hitter will be thick and somewhat gooey.

7. Pour the hitter into the oiled or lined dish and place it on the stove.

8. Bake for 40 minutes. The bread will rise essentially on the stove.

9. Remove from the stove and let it cool totally around 1 to 2 hours. The bread will sink a few and that is OK. When the bread has cooled, run the sharp edge of a blade around the edges of the dish to transfer the portion. Cut into 12 even cuts.

Nutrition:

- Calories: 20
- Carbohydrates: 8 g
- Net Carbohydrates: 2.5 g
- Fiber: 4.5 g
- Fat: 6 g
- Protein: 8 g

Easy Cloud Bread

Preparation Time: 5 minutes
Cooking time: 18 minutes
Servings: 7

Ingredients:

- 3 eggs
- 3 teaspoons of coconut cream spoon from a refrigerated container of full-fat coconut milk
- 1/2 teaspoon preparing powder

Discretionary Ingredients:

- ocean salt
- dark pepper and rosemary or whatever seasonings you like!

Directions:

1. Firstly, prep everything. When you start going, you'll have to move rapidly so have everything convenient. Preheat the stove to 325°F and place a rack in the center. Line a heating sheet with material paper and put it in a safe spot. Get your devices: hand blender (you can use a stand blender as well, yet I see it as better for whipping egg whites so I can remain in charge), all ingredients, any extra

seasonings, two blending bowls (the larger one ought to be used for egg whites), a big spoon to scoop and drop the bread with.

2. Using a full-fat jar of coconut milk that has been refrigerated medium-term or for few hours, spoon out the top coconut cream and add to the smaller bowl.

3. Separate eggs into the two dishes, adding the yolk to the bowl with the cream, and be careful not to let the yolk get into the whites in the bigger bowl.

4. Using a hand blender, beat the yolk and cream together first until pleasant and smooth, ensure there are no clusters of coconut left.

5. Wash your whisks well and dry them.

6. Add the preparing powder into the whites and start beating on medium with the hand blender for a couple of minutes, moving around and you'll see it get firmer. Keep blending for a couple of minutes, you need to get it as thick as you can with firm pinnacles. The thicker the better. Simply don't over-do it. When you can stop and dunk the speeds in deserting tops, you're prepared.

7. Quickly and cautiously, add the yolk-coconut blend into the whites, stirring with a spatula, cautious not to empty excessively. Keep blending until everything is very much consolidated, yet soft.

8. Now you can get your spoon and start dropping your hitter down on the heating sheet. Keep blending as fast and cautiously as you can, or it will begin to liquefy. They should look cushiony.

9. Steadily add your heating sheet to the center rack in the stove and bake for approx. 20-25 minutes. You ought to have the option to scoop them up with your spatula and see a soft top and a level base. Store in the ice chest for about a week or freeze.

Nutrition:

- Calories: 300
- Carbohydrates: 4 g
- Net Carbohydrates: 2.5 g
- Fiber: 4.5 g
- Fat: 8 g
- Protein: 8 g

Keto Breadsticks

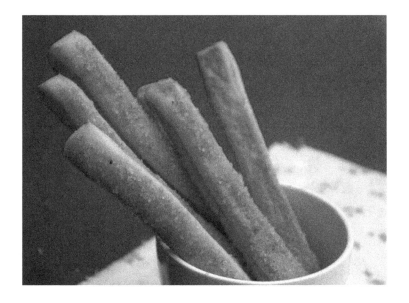

Preparation Time: 6 minutes

Cooking time: 30 minutes

Servings: 15

Ingredients:

<u>Bread Stick Base</u>

- 2 cups mozzarella cheese (~8 oz.)
- 3/4 cup almond flour
- 1 tablespoon psyllium husk powder
- 3 tablespoons cream cheese (~1.5 oz.)
- 1 large egg

- 1 teaspoon preparing powder

Italian Style
- 2 tablespoons Italian seasoning
- 1 teaspoon salt
- 1 teaspoon pepper

Extra Cheesy
- 1 teaspoon garlic powder
- 1 teaspoon onion powder
- 3 oz. Cheddar cheese
- 1/4 cup Parmesan cheese
- Cinnamon sugar
- 3 tablespoon spread
- 6 tablespoon swerve sweetener
- 2 tablespoon cinnamon

Directions:
- Pre-heat stove to 400°F. Combine egg and cream cheddar until somewhat blended. In another bowl, mix all the dry ingredients.
- Measure out the mozzarella cheddar and microwave in 20-second interims until sizzling.
- Add the egg, cream cheddar, and dry ingredients into the mozzarella cheddar and combine.

- Using your hands, knead the batter and press level on a Silpat.
- Transfer the batter to some thwart so you can use a pizza shaper on it, then season the mixture with the flavorings you like.
- Bake 13-15 minutes on top rack until fresh.
- Serve while warm!

Nutrition:
- Calories: 60
- Carbohydrates: 4 g
- Net Carbohydrates: 2.5 g
- Fiber: 4.5 g
- Fat: 6 g
- Protein: 4 g

Bagels Bread for keto diet

Preparation Time: 5 minutes

Cooking time: 17 minutes

Servings: 6

Ingredients:

- 1 cup (120 g) of almond flour
- 1/4 cup (28 g) of coconut flour
- 1 tablespoon (7 g) of psyllium husk powder
- 1 teaspoon (2 g) of preparing powder
- 1 teaspoon (3 g) of garlic powder
- Pinch salt
- 2 medium eggs (88 g)
- 2 teaspoons (10 ml) of white wine vinegar
- 2 ½ tablespoons (38 ml) of ghee, dissolved
- 1 tablespoon (15 ml) of olive oil
- 1 teaspoon (5 g) of sesame seeds

Directions:

1. Preheat the stove to 320°F (160°C).
2. Combine the almond flour, coconut flour, psyllium husk powder, preparing powder, garlic powder, and salt in a bowl.

3. In a different bowl, whisk the eggs and vinegar together. Gradually dip in the dissolved ghee (which ought not to be steaming hot) and speed in well.

4. Add the wet blend to the dry blend and use a wooden spoon to mix well. Leave to sit for 2-3 minutes.

5. Divide the blend into 4 equivalent measured bits. With your hands, shape the blend into a round shape and place it onto a plate fixed with material paper. Use a little spoon or apple corer to make the middle gap.

6. Brush the tops with olive oil and spread out the sesame seeds. Cook in the broiler for 20-25 minutes until cooked through. Allow to cool marginally before getting a charge out of!

Nutrition:

- Calories: 10
- Carbohydrates: 1 g
- Net Carbohydrates: 1.5 g
- Fiber: 2.5 g
- Fat: 8 g
- Protein: 9 g

Cranberry Jalapeño "Cornbread" Muffins

Preparation Time: 6 minutes

Cooking time: 19 minutes

Servings: 8

Ingredients:

- 1 cup coconut flour
- 1/3 cup Swerve Sweetener or another erythritol
- 1 teaspoon heating powder
- 1/2 teaspoon salt
- 7 large eggs, softly beaten
- 1 cup unsweetened almond milk
- 1/2 cup margarine, softened or avocado oil
- 1/2 teaspoon vanilla
- 1 cup crisp cranberries cut down the middle
- 3 teaspoons minced jalapeño peppers
- 1 jalapeño, seeds evacuated, cut into 12 cuts, to decorate

Directions:

1. Preheat stove to 325°F and oil a biscuit tin well or line with paper liners.

2. In a medium bowl, whisk together coconut flour, sugar, heating powder, and salt. Separate any clusters with the rear of a fork.

3. Stir in eggs softened spread and almond milk and whisk. Mix in vanilla concentrate and keep on mixing until the blend is smooth and very much joined. Mix in slashed cranberries and jalapeños.

4. Divide player equally among arranged biscuit cups and place one cut of jalapeño over each.

5. Bake 25 to 30 minutes or until tops are set. Let them cool for 10 minutes in access dish; then move to a wire rack to cool totally.

Nutrition:

- Cal: 10
- Carbohydrates: 4 g
- Net Carbohydrates: 2.5 g
- Fiber: 4.5 g
- Fat: 8 g
- Protein: 8 g

Zucchini Bread with Walnuts

Preparation Time: 11 minutes

Cooking time: 30 minutes

Servings: 12

Ingredients:

- 1 large egg
- 1 tablespoon almond flour
- 1 tablespoon psyllium husk powder
- ¼ teaspoon preparing powder
- ¼ teaspoon cream of tartar
- 1 tablespoon chicken soup
- 1 tablespoon dissolved spread

Directions:

1. Crack an egg into a mug and pour in the dissolved spread. Mix together well until eggs are lighter in shading.
2. Add the rest of the ingredients and blend well. You should wind up with a somewhat raw substance.
3. Microwave for 60-75 seconds, contingent upon the wattage of microwave (it will puff up in the mug, and lessen incredibly in size on you take it out).
4. Slice down the middle and sauté in the spread.

Nutrition:

- Calories: 100
- Carbs: 4 g
- Net Carbohydrates: 2.5 g
- Fiber: 4.5 g
- Fat: 8 g
- Protein: 9 g

Buttery & Soft Skillet Flatbread

Preparation Time: 9 minutes

Cooking time: 22 minutes

Servings: 8

Ingredients:

- 1 cup almond flour
- 2 teaspoons coconut flour
- 2 teaspoons xanthan gum
- 1/2 teaspoon heating powder
- 1/2 teaspoon falk salt
- 1 whole egg + 1 egg white
- 1 teaspoon water
- 1 teaspoon oil for searing
- 1 teaspoon liquefied butter-for slathering

Directions:

1. Whisk together the dry ingredients (flours, thickener, preparing powder, salt) until very much consolidated.
2. Add the egg and egg white and beat tenderly into the flour to mix. The mixture will start to frame.
3. Add the tablespoon of water and start to work the batter to permit the flour and thickener to retain the dampness.

4. Divide the batter into 4 equal parts and press each area out with stick wrap.
5. Heat a big skillet over medium warmth and add oil.
6. Fry every flatbread for around 1 min on each side.
7. Brush with margarine (while hot) and garnish with salt and cleaved parsley.

Nutrition:

- Calories: 50
- Carbohydrates: 10 g
- Net Carbohydrates: 6 g
- Fiber: 4.5 g
- Fat: 8 g
- Protein: 9 g

Blueberry English muffin Bread Loaf

Preparation Time: 4 minutes

Cooking time: 14 minutes

Servings: 5

Ingredients:

- 1/2 cup almond spread or cashew or nutty spread
- 1/4 cup spread ghee or coconut oil
- 1/2 cup almond flour
- 1/2 teaspoon salt
- 2 teaspoons preparing powder
- 1/2 cup almond milk unsweetened
- 5 eggs, beaten
- 1/2 cup blueberries

Directions:

1. Preheat stove to 350 °F.
2. In a microwavable bowl, melt nut margarine and spread together for 30 seconds, mix until joined well.
3. In a big bowl, whisk almond flour, salt, and heating powder together. Empty the nut spread blend into the big bowl and mix to consolidate.
4. Whisk the almond milk and eggs together, then fill the bowl and mix well.

5. Drop-in new blueberries or break separated solidified blueberries and tenderly mix into the hitter.
6. Line a portion dish with material paper and daintily also oil the material paper.
7. Pour the hitter into the portion dish and cook for 45 minutes or until a toothpick inserted in the center comes out dry.
8. Cool for around 30 minutes, and then remove from the container.
9. Slice and toast each cut before serving.

Nutrition:

- Calories: 50
- Carbohydrates: 4g
- Net Carbohydrates: 2.5 g
- Fiber: 4.5 g
- Fat: 7 g
- Protein: 6g

Low-Carb Garlic & Herb Focaccia Bread

Preparation Time: 10 minutes

Cooking time: 25 minutes

Servings: 7

Ingredients:

- 1 cup almond flour
- ¼ cup coconut flour
- ½ teaspoon xanthan gum
- 1 teaspoon garlic powder
- 1 teaspoon flaky salt
- ½ teaspoon heating soda
- ½ teaspoon heating powder

Wet Ingredients:

- 2 eggs
- 1 teaspoon lemon juice
- 2 teaspoons olive oil + 2 teaspoons of olive oil to sprinkle
- Top with italian seasoning and tons of flaky salt!

Directions:

1. Heat broiler to 350 °F and line a preparing plate or 8-inch round dish with the material.

2. Whisk together the dry ingredients, ensuring there are no knots.
3. Beat the egg, lemon squeeze, and oil until combined.
4. Mix the wet and the dry together, whisking, and scoop the mixture into your dish.
5. Make sure not to blend the wet and dry until you are prepared to place the bread in the broiler on the grounds that the raising response starts once it is blended!!!
6. Smooth the top and edges with a spatula dunked in water (or your hands), then use your finger to dimple the batter. Try not to be hesitant to dive deep into the dimples! Once more, a little water prevents it from sticking.
7. Bake secured for around 10 minutes. Sprinkle with olive oil. Heat for an extra 10-15 minutes until it is dark-colored.
8. Top with increasingly flaky salt, olive oil (discretionary), a scramble of Italian flavoring, and crisp basil. Let it cool totally before cutting for an ideal surface!!

Nutrition:
- Calories: 80
- Carbohydrates: 16 g
- Net Carbohydrates: 2.5 g
- Fiber: 8.5 g
- Fat: 7 g
- Protein: 8 g

Chocolate Zucchini Bread

Preparation Time: 5 minutes

Cooking time: 20 minutes

Servings: 8

Ingredients:

- 1 ½ cup almond flour (170g)
- 1/4 cup unsweetened cocoa powder (25g)
- 1 ½ teaspoon heating pop
- 2 teaspoons ground cinnamon
- 1/4 teaspoon ocean salt
- 1/2 cup sugar-free precious stone sugar (Monk natural product or erythritol) (100g) or coconut sugar whenever refined sugar-free

Wet Ingredients:

- 1 cup zucchini, finely ground measure pressed, dispose of juice/fluid if there is a few - around 2 little zucchini
- 1 large egg
- 1/4 cup + 2 tablespoons canned coconut cream 100ml
- 1/4 cup additional virgin coconut oil, softened, 60ml
- 1 teaspoon vanilla concentrate
- 1 teaspoon apple juice vinegar

<u>Filling - discretionary</u>

- 1/2 cup sugar-free chocolate chips
- 1/2 cup cleaved pecans or nuts you like

Directions:

1. Preheat broiler to 180°C (375°F). Line a heating portion skillet (9 inches x 5 inches) with material paper. Put in a safe spot.

2. Remove the two furthest points of the zucchinis, keep the skin on.

3. Finely mash the zucchini using a vegetable grater. Measure the amount required in an estimation cup. Ensure you press/pack them solidly for an exact measure and to crush out any fluid from the ground zucchini, I, as a rule, don't have any! In the event that you do, dispose of the fluid or keep it for another formula.

4. In a large blending bowl, mix all the dry ingredients together: almond flour, unsweetened cocoa powder, sugar-free precious stone sugar, cinnamon, ocean salt, and heating pop. Put in a safe spot. Add all the wet ingredients into the dry ingredients— ground zucchini, coconut oil, coconut cream, vanilla, egg, apple juice vinegar.

5. Stir to combine every one of the ingredients together.

6. Stir in the cleaved nuts and sugar-free chocolate chips.

7. Transfer the chocolate bread player into the readied portion container.

8. Bake 50 −55 minutes, you might need to cover the bread portion with a bit of foil after 40 minutes to maintain a strategic distance from the top to turn brown excessively. That is up to you.

9. The bread will remain somewhat wet in the center and harden after completely chilled off.

Nutrition:

- Calories: 300
- Carbohydrates: 7 g
- Net Carbohydrates: 11.5 g
- Fiber: 4.5 g
- Fat: 13 g
- Protein: 1 g

Banana Almond Bread

Preparation Time: 20 minutes

Cooking time: 2 hours

Total Time: 2 hours 20 minutes

Servings: 12 slices

Ingredients:

- 2 large eggs
- 1/3 cup butter, unsalted
- 1/8 cup almond milk, unsweetened
- 2 medium mashed bananas
- 1 1/3 cups almond flour
- 0.63 teaspoon Stevia extract sugar
- 1 ¼ teaspoons Baking powder
- ½ teaspoon baking soda
- ½ teaspoon salt
- ½ cup chopped nuts

Directions:

1. Prepare all the ingredients.
2. Ensure all ingredients are at room temperature. Place the butter, eggs, milk, and mashed bananas in the bread bucket.

3. In a mixing bowl, combine all the dry ingredients and mix well.

4. Pour the dry ingredients into the bread bucket.

5. Set the bread machine in Quick Bread, then close the lid and let it cook until the machine beeps.

6. Cool the bread before slicing and serving.

Nutrition:

- Calories: 147
- Calories from fat: 90
- Total Fat: 10 g
- Total Carbohydrates: 13 g
- Net Carbohydrates: 12 g
- Protein: 2 g

Low-Carb Bread

Preparation Time: 5 minutes

Cooking time: 31 minutes

Servings: 1

Ingredients:

- 2 tablespoons almond flour
- 1/2 tablespoon coconut flour
- 1/4 teaspoon heating powder
- 1 egg
- 1/2 tablespoon liquefied margarine or ghee
- 1 tablespoon unsweetened milk of decision

Directions:

1. Blend all ingredients in a little bowl and whisk until smooth.
2. Oil a 3×3-inch glass microwave-safe bowl or shape with spread, ghee, or coconut oil
3. Empty your blend into your well-lubed bowl or shape and microwave on High for 90 seconds.
4. Cautiously remove your bread from the glass dish or shape.
5. Cut, toast, and liquefy spread on top, whenever wanted.

Nutrition:

- Calories: 270
- Fat: 15 g
- Fiber: 3 g
- Carbohydrates: 5 g
- Protein: 9 g

Low-Carb "Rye" Bread

Preparation Time: 22 minutes

Cooking time: 1 hour

Servings: 5

Dry Ingredients:

- 2 pressed cups ground flaxseed (300g/10.6 oz.)
- 1 cup coconut flour (120g/4.2 oz.)
- 2 tablespoons caraway seeds (or rosemary)
- 1 tablespoon + 1 teaspoon heating powder (I utilized my very own sans gluten preparing blend: 1 teaspoon heating soft drink added to the dry blend + 2 teaspoon cream of tartar added to the egg whites)
- 1 tablespoon Erythritol (10g/0.4 oz.) or 5 drops fluid stevia
- 1/4 cup ground chia seeds (32g/1.1 oz.) or 1 tablespoon (thickener isn't paleo-accommodating)
- 1 teaspoon salt or more to taste (pink Himalayan stone salt)

Wet Ingredients:

- 8 eggs (unfenced, natural, or "omega-3" eggs), isolated
- 1/2 cup relaxed yet not dissolved grass-encouraged ghee or spread or 1/2 cup additional virgin olive oil (110g/3.9 oz.)

59

- 2 tablespoons toasted sesame oil (together with the caraway seeds, this is the key fixing!)
- 1/3 cup apple juice vinegar (80 ml/2.7 fl oz.)
- 1 cup warm water (240 ml/8 fl oz.)

Directions:

1. Move the broiler rack to the middle of the stove, and preheat to 175 °C/350 °F. Add the dry ingredients to a big bowl and whisk together (ground flaxseed, coconut flour, caraway, heating pop, Erythritol, salt, and thickener or ground chia seeds). It is particularly hard to uniformly fit the thickener (or ground chia seeds).

2. Separate the egg yolks from the egg whites and keep the egg whites aside. Add relaxed ghee or spread and toasted sesame oil into the egg yolks.

3. Note: Although the first formula doesn't request isolating the eggs, I found that doing so makes the bread more "feathery".

4. "Cream" the egg yolks and the ghee (spread or olive oil) until smooth. In a different bowl, whisk the egg whites until they make delicate pinnacles and "fix" them with the cream of tartar.

5. Add the dry blend to the bowl with the egg yolk blend and mix well. It's a thick player and will meet up gradually. Set aside and try to ensure everything is completely blended.

6. Add the vinegar and blend in well.
7. Add warm water and mix until combined.
8. Add the egg whites and tenderly crease them in. Do whatever it takes not to empty the player totally.
9. Oil a big portion container with some ghee or margarine and add the player. Smooth the player out equally in the skillet and "cut" it on top using a spatula to make a wave impact.
10. Note: If you use a silicon portion container, you won't have to oil it.
11. Prepare for a roughly 50-an hour (relies upon the stove). Then when the bread is prepared, remove from portion dish to a cooling rack, and let it cool completely.

Nutrition:
- Calories: 270
- Fat: 15 g
- Fiber: 3 g
- Carbohydrates: 5 g
- Protein: 9 g

Microwave Mug Bread

Preparation Time: 8 minutes

Cooking time: 15 minutes

Servings: 10

Ingredients:

- 1 egg
- 1 teaspoon coconut flour
- 1/4 teaspoon preparing powder
- 1 teaspoon spread

Directions:

1. Crack your egg into a microwave-safe ramekin or glass mug and beat it with a fork.

2. Add 1 tablespoon of coconut flour and 1/4 teaspoon of preparing powder to the egg, then microwave around 1 tablespoon of margarine in a different microwave-safe dish and add it to the blend. Then blend it well with the fork. The blend ought to be very thick.

3. Pop the dish into the microwave for 90 seconds and be cautious when removing it as it will be hot. In the event that the bread doesn't fall directly out when you flip your dish over, pull the sides away with a fork or margarine

blade and your bread should come directly out. Cut it down the middle and trim the sides if needed.

Nutrition:

- Calories: 20
- Carbohydrates: 4 g
- Net Carbohydrates: 2.5 g
- Fiber: 4.5 g
- Fat: 6 g
- Protein: 7 g

Low-Carb Cauliflower Bread

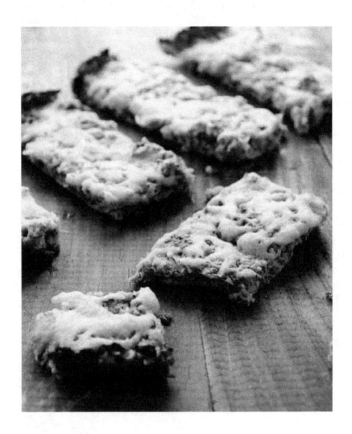

Preparation Time: 20 minutes

Cooking time: 45 min

Servings: 8

Ingredients:

- 2 cups almond flour
- 5 eggs
- ¼ cup psyllium husk

- 1 cup cauliflower rice

Directions:

1. Preheat broiler to 350 °F.
2. Line a portion skillet with material paper or coconut oil cooking shower. Put in a safe spot.
3. In a big bowl or food processor, blend the almond flour and psyllium husk.
4. Beat in the eggs on high for as long as two minutes.
5. Blend in the cauliflower rice and mix well.
6. Empty the cauliflower blend into the portion skillet.
7. Heat for as long as 55 minutes.

Nutrition:

- Calories: 21

- Fat: 4.7 g

- Carbohydrates: 44.2 g

- Protein: 0 g

Low Carb Microwave Hamburger Bread

Preparation Time: 7 minutes

Cooking time: 15 minutes

Servings: 8

Ingredients:

Bagels:

- ¾ cup (68 g) almond flour
- 1 teaspoon thickener
- 1 large egg
- 1 ½ cups ground mozzarella
- 2 tablespoons cream cheddar
- 1 tablespoon spread, dissolved
- Sesame seeds to taste

Fillings

- 2 tablespoons pesto
- 2 tablespoons cream cheddar
- 1 cup arugula leaves
- 6 cuts flame-broiled streaky bacon

Directions:

1. Preheat stove to 390°F.

2. In a bowl, combine the almond flour and thickener. Then add the egg and blend together until well combined. Put in a safe spot. It will resemble a sticky ball.

3. In a pot, over medium-low warmth gradually, melt the cream cheddar and mozzarella together and remove from heat once liquefied. This should also be possible in the microwave.

4. Add your melted cheddar blend to the almond flour blend and mix until well combined. The Mozzarella mix will stick in somewhat of a ball yet don't stress, endure with it. It will all, in the end, combine well. It's hard to get the Xanthan gum fused through the cheddar blend. On the off chance that the mixture gets too intense to even think about working, place in the microwave for 10-20 seconds to warm and rehash until you have something that takes after batter.

5. Split your batter into 3 pieces and fold into round logs. On the off chance that you have a doughnut dish place your logs into the container. If not, make hovers with each log and consolidate and place it on a heating plate. Try to ensure you have decent circles. The other method to do this is to make a ball and straighten somewhat on the heating plate and cut a hover out of the center on the off chance that you have a little cutout.

6. Melt your spread and brush over the highest point of your bagels and sprinkle sesame seeds or you're fixing of decision. The spread should enable the seeds to stick. Garlic and onion powder or cheddar causes decent increases, in the event that you have them for flavorful bagels.

7. Place bagels on the stove for around 18 minutes. Watch out for them. The tops ought to go brilliant dark-colored.

8. Take the bagels out of the stove and permit cooling.

9. If you like your bagels toasted, cut them down the middle longwise and place them back on the stove until marginally brilliant and toasty.

10. Spread bagel with creamy Cheddar, spread in pesto, add a couple of arugula leaves, and top with your fresh bacon (or your desired filling)

Nutrition:

- Calories: 90
- Carbohydrates: 4 g
- Net Carbohidrates: 2.5 g
- Fiber: 4.5 g
- Fat: 8 g
- Protein: 8 g

Microwave Flax Bread

Preparation Time: 7 minutes

Cooking time: 25 min

Servings: 13

Ingredients:

- 1 teaspoon spread
- 1 large egg
- 4 teaspoons ground flaxseed
- 1/2 teaspoon preparing powder

Directions:

1. Add 1 tablespoon of spread to a microwave-safe ramekin and liquefy it in the microwave (10-20 seconds). Split your egg into the dish with the margarine and beat it with a fork.

2. Add 4 tablespoon of ground flaxseed, 1/2 teaspoon of preparing powder, and a spot of salt. Then blend it well with the fork. The blend ought to be thick, so shake the dish around a piece to even it out.

3. Pop the dish into the microwave for 2 minutes and be cautious when removing it as it will be hot. On the off chance that the bread doesn't fall directly out when you flip your dish over, pull the sides away with a fork or margarine

blade and your bread should come directly out. Cool it on a rack and cut it down the middle.

Nutrition:

- Calories: 30
- Carbohydrates: 4 g
- Net Carbohydrates: 2.5 g
- Fiber: 4.5 g
- Fat: 3 g
- Protein: 1 g

Keto Milk and Honey Breakfast Loaf

Preparation Time: 2 hours

Cooking time: 10 minutes

Total Time: 2 hours 10 minutes

Servings: 18 slices

Ingredients:

- 1 cup + 1 tablespoon almond milk, unsweetened
- 3 tablespoons honey
- 3 tablespoons melted butter
- 1 ½ teaspoons salts
- 3 cups almond flour
- 2 teaspoons active dry yeast

Directions:

1. Put all ingredients in the bread bucket as listed in the ingredient list.
2. Select the Basic cycle on your bread machine setting, close the lid then press Start.
3. Once the loaf is ready, remove it from the machine and place it in a cooling rack.
4. Slice and serve with your favorite spread.

Nutrition:

- Calories: 39
- Calories from fat: 27
- Total Fat: 3 g
- Total Carbohydrates: 3 g
- Net Carbohydrates: 3 g
- Protein: 1 g

Low Carb Flax Bread

Preparation Time: 10 minutes

Cooking time: 24 minutes

Servings: 8

Ingredients:

- 200 g ground flax seeds
- ½ cup psyllium husk powder
- 1 tablespoon heating powder
- 1 ½ cups soy protein separate
- ¼ cup granulated Stevia
- 2 teaspoons salt
- 7 large egg whites
- 1 big entire egg
- 3 tablespoons margarine
- ¾ cup water

Directions:

1. Preheat broiler to 350 ° F.
2. Mix psyllium husk, heating powder, protein disengage, sugar, and salt together in a bowl.

3. In a different bowl, blend egg, egg whites, margarine, and water together. On the off chance that you are including concentrates or syrups, add them here.
4. Slowly add wet ingredients to dry ingredients and combine.
5. Grease your bread dish with a spread or splash.
6. Add the blend to the bread dish
7. Bake 15-20 minutes until set.

Nutrition:

- Calories: 20

- Carbohydrates: 5 g

- Net Carbohydrates: 5.5 g

- Fiber: 8.5

- Fat: 13 g

- Protein: 10 g

Low Carb Focaccia Bread

Preparation Time: 10 minutes

Cooking time: 25 minutes

Servings: 12

Ingredients:

- 1 cup almond flour
- 1 cup flaxseed feast
- 7 large eggs
- ¼ cup olive oil
- 1 ½ tablespoons heating powder
- 2 teaspoons minced garlic
- 1 teaspoon salt
- 1 teaspoon rosemary
- 1 teaspoon red bean stew chips

Directions:

1. Preheat your broiler to 350°F.
2. In a blending bowl, add all the dry ingredients and blend well.
3. Start adding garlic and 2 eggs one after another, blending in with a hand blender to get a firm mixture.

4. Add olive oil last, blending it well until everything is combined. The more aerated the mix turns into, the more "cushy" your bread will turn into.

5. Put every one of your ingredients into a lubed 9x9 heating dish, smooth out with a spatula.

6. Bake for 25 minutes.

7. Let it cool for 10 minutes and remove it from the lubed heating dish.

8. Cut into squares and cut the squares down the middle. Add whatever you'd prefer to the center!

Nutrition:

- Calories: 50
- Carbohydrates: 4 g
- Net Carbohydrates: 2.5 g
- Fiber: 4.5 g
- Fat: 8 g
- Protein: 8 g

Cinnamon Almond Flour Bread

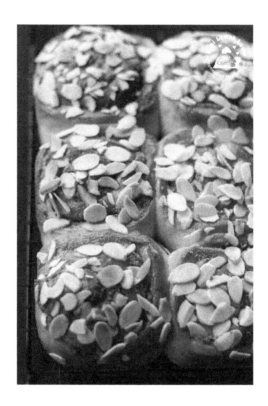

Preparation Time: 7 minutes

Cooking time: 18 minutes

Servings: 9

Ingredients:

- 2 cups fine whitened almond flour (I utilize Bob's, Red Mill)
- 2 teaspoons coconut flour
- 1/2 teaspoon ocean salt

- 1 teaspoon heating pop
- 1/4 cup Flaxseed supper or chia dinner (ground chia or flaxseed; see notes for how to make your own)
- 5 eggs and 1 egg white whisked together
- 1.5 teaspoon Apple juice vinegar or lemon juice
- 2 teaspoon maple syrup or nectar
- 2–3 teaspoons of explained spread (dissolved) or Coconut oil; separated. Vegetarian margarine likewise works
- 1 teaspoon cinnamon in addition to extra for fixing
- Optional: chia seed to sprinkle on the top before preparing

Directions:

1. Preheat stove to 350°F. Line an 8×4 bread dish with material paper at the base and oil the sides.
2. In a big bowl, combine your almond flour, coconut flour, salt, preparing pop, flaxseed feast or chia supper, and 1/2 tablespoon of cinnamon.
3. In another little bowl, whisk together your eggs and egg white. Then add the maple syrup (or nectar), apple juice vinegar, and melted margarine (1.5 to 2 teaspoons).
4. Mix wet ingredients into dry. Make sure to remove any bunches that may have left from the almond flour or coconut flour.
5. Pour hitter into your lubed portion container.

6. Bake at 350° for 30-35 minutes, until a toothpick inserted in the middle comes out clean. Mine too around 35 minutes yet I am at elevation.

7. Remove from the broiler.

8. Next, whisk together the other 1 to 2 teaspoon of softened margarine (or oil) and blend it in with 1/2 teaspoon of cinnamon. Brush this over cinnamon almond flour bread.

9. Cool and serve or store for some other time.

Nutrition:

- Calories: 200
- Carbohydrates: 4 g
- Net Carbohydrates: 10.5 g
- Fiber: 4.5 g
- Fat: 8 g
- Protein: 8 g

Ciabatta Bread for keto diet

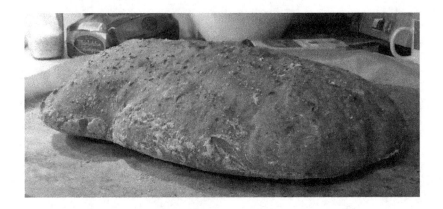

Preparation Time: 120 minutes

Cooking time: 40 minutes

Total Time: 2 hours 40 minutes

Servings: 6 slices

Ingredients:

- 1 cup + 2 tablespoons warm water, divided
- 1 teaspoon sugar
- 2 ¼ teaspoons dry active yeast
- 1 cup vital wheat gluten
- 1 cup superfine almond flour
- ¼ cup flax seed meal
- ¾ teaspoon salt
- 1 ½ teaspoons baking powder

- 3 tablespoons extra virgin olive oil
- 1 tablespoon melted butter

Directions:

1. In a bowl, add ½-cup warm water, sugar, and yeast. Cover and let it sit for 10 minutes or until frothy.

2. In your bread machine bucket, add the yeast mixture, the remaining ½ cup, and 2 tablespoons Water and olive oil. Add flour, flaxseed, salt, and baking powder. Place the bread bucket back in the bread machine and close the lid.

3. Set the bread machine to Dough cycle, close the lid, then press the Start button. After 10 minutes, stop the bread machine. You will have a very sticky dough.

4. Pour the dough on a floured surface and divide it in half before rolling into a tube-like shape (about 2.5 x 7 inches). Place the cut dough on a greased cookie sheet.

5. Preheat your oven for 2 to 3 minutes at 110 °F. Turn the oven off and place the dough inside to rise for 1 hour. After 1 hour, you should have about 3.5 x 8 inches raised dough.

6. Preheat your oven at 350 °F to start baking.

7. Brush your raised dough with melted butter, then bake for 15 minutes. Take out of the oven and brush once more with butter before returning inside the oven —for another 10 to 15 minutes until the dough's internal temperature reaches 200 °F.

8. Once done, let the loaf cool for 1 hour before slicing.

9. Serve with scrambled egg or your favorite jam.

Nutrition:

- Calories: 286
- Calories from fat: 171
- Total Fat: 19 g
- Total Carbohydrates: 9 g
- Net Carbohydrates: 5 g
- Protein: 21 g

Healthy Low Carb Bread

Preparation Time: 15 minutes

Cooking time: 35 minutes

Servings: 8

Ingredients:

- 2/3 cup coconut flour
- 2/3 cup coconut oil (softened not melted)
- 9 eggs
- 2 teaspoons cream of tartar
- ¾ teaspoon xanthan gum
- 1 teaspoon baking soda
- ¼ teaspoon salt

Directions:

1. Preheat the oven to 350°F.
2. Grease a loaf pan with 1 to 2 teaspoon melted coconut oil and place in the freezer to harden.
3. Add eggs into a bowl and mix for 2 minutes with a hand mixer.
4. Add coconut oil into the eggs and mix.
5. Add dry ingredients to a second bowl and whisk until mixed.

6. Add the dry ingredients into the egg mixture and mix on low speed with a hand mixer until dough is formed and the mixture is added.

7. Add the dough into the prepared loaf pan, transfer it into the preheated oven, and bake for 35 minutes.

8. Take out loaf pan from the oven.

9. Cool, slice, and serve.

Nutrition:

- Calories: 229
- Fat: 25.5 g
- Carbohydrates: 6.5 g
- Protein: 8.5 g

Super Seed Bread

Preparation Time: 5 minutes

Cooking time: 22 minutes

Servings: 7

Ingredients:

- 2/3 cup entire psyllium husk
- 1/4 cup chia seeds
- 1/4 cup pumpkin seeds
- 1/4 cup hemp or sunflower seeds
- 1 teaspoon ground sesame seeds or ground flaxseeds 1 teaspoon preparing powder
- 1/4 teaspoon salt
- 2 teaspoons coconut oil
- 1 1/4 cups fluid egg
- 1/2 cup unsweetened almond milk

Directions:

- In a large blending bowl, add every single dry ingredient and blend well. You can make your own ground sesame seeds by mixing them until they're a fine powder.
- Melt the coconut oil in the microwave (around 30 seconds), add it to the dry blend and mix well. Then add

1/4 cup fluid egg whites and 1/2 cup unsweetened almond milk. Blend well and let the blend sit for 10-15 minutes while you preheat your stove to 325° F.

- Wet some material paper under warm water and shake it off, then press it into a 9" x 5" bread tin. Add the blend and press it into the edges of the tin. You can likewise add some additional seeds to the highest point of the blend here. Trim enough material paper and put it on the stove for 70 minutes.

- Slice the whole portion and let it cool on a drying rack. This bread can empty if not cut at the earliest opportunity and leave it to cool on a rack.

Nutrition:
- Calories: 70
- Carbohidrates: 4 g
- Net Carbohydrates: 2.5 g
- Fiber: 4.5 g
- Fat: 8 g
- Protein: 8 g

Pumpkin Pecan Bread

Preparation Time: 10 minutes

Cooking time: 3 hours

Servings: 1 loaf, 16

Ingredients:

- 1/2 cup milk
- 1/2 cup canned pumpkin
- 1 egg
- 2 tablespoons margarine or butter, cut up
- 3 cups bread flour
- 3 tablespoons packed brown sugar
- 3/4 teaspoon salt
- 1/4 teaspoon ground nutmeg
- 1/4 teaspoon ground ginger
- 1/8 teaspoon ground cloves
- 1 teaspoon active dry yeast or bread machine yeast
- 3/4 cup coarsely chopped pecans

Direction:

1. Add all ingredients to the machine pan.
2. Select Basic cycle.

Nutrition:

- Calories: 159
- Total fat: 6 g (1 g sat. fat)
- Carbohydrates: 23 g
- Fiber:1 g
- Protein: 4 g

Delicious Carrot Cake

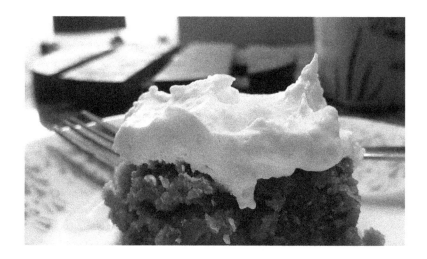

Preparation Time: 15 minutes

Cooking time: 55 minutes

Servings: 6

Ingredients:

- 2 large eggs
- 1/2 cup carrots, grated
- 1 teaspoon vanilla
- 2 tablespoons coconut oil, melted
- 3 tablespoons heavy cream
- ¼ teaspoon nutmeg
- ½ teaspoon cinnamon
- 1 teaspoon baking powder

- 2/3 cup Swerve
- 1 cup almond flour

For Frosting:
- 1 tablespoon heavy cream
- ½ teaspoon vanilla
- 2 teaspoons fresh lemon juice
- 3 tablespoons swerve
- 4 oz cream cheese, softened

Directions:

1. Take a cake pan that fits into the instant pot, spray with cooking spray, and set aside.
2. Drain excess liquid from grated carrots.
3. In a mixing bowl, mix together almond flour, grated carrots, vanilla, coconut oil, heavy cream, eggs, nutmeg, cinnamon, baking powder, and swerve using a hand mixer until well combined.
4. Pour batter into the prepared cake pan and cover the pan with foil.
5. Add 1 2/3 cup of water to the instant pot, then place steamer rack into the pot.
6. Place cake pan on the steamer rack.
7. Seal the instant pot with the lid and select manual high pressure and set the timer for 45 minutes.

8. Allow releasing pressure naturally for 10 minutes, then release using the Quick release method.

9. Open the lid carefully and remove the cake pan from the pot. Let the cake cool for 30 minutes.

10. Meanwhile, make the frosting. In a large bowl, add heavy cream, vanilla, lemon juice, swerve, and cream cheese and beat using a hand mixer until creamy.

11. Once the cake is cool completely, then frost the cake using prepared cream.

12. Cut cake into slices and serve.

Nutrition:

- Calories. 289
- Fat: 25.9 g
- Carbohydrates: 10.9 g
- Protein: 7.9 g

Purple Yam Pancakes

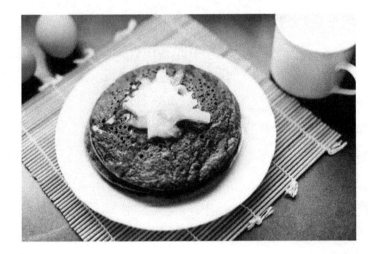

Preparation Time: 5 minutes

Cooking time: 10 minutes

Servings: 4

Ingredients:
- ½ Cup coconut flour
- 4 eggs
- 1 cup coconut milk
- 1 teaspoon guar gum
- ½ teaspoon baking powder
- 1 tablespoon coconut oil
- ¼ cup purple yam puree

Directions:

1. Mix all ingredients in a blender.
2. Preheat a skillet and coat with non-stick spray.
3. Ladle in the batter and cook for 1-2 minutes per side.

Nutrition:

- Kcal per serve: 347
- Fat: 31 g (76%)
- Protein: 11 g. (13%)
- Carbohidrates: 9 g (11%)

Almond Coconut Cake

Preparation Time: 10 minutes

Cooking time: 50 minutes

Servings: 8

Ingredients:

- 2 eggs, lightly beaten
- ½ cup heavy cream
- ¼ cup coconut oil, melted
- 1 teaspoon cinnamon
- 1 teaspoon baking powder
- 1/3 cup Swerve
- ½ cup unsweetened shredded coconut
- 1 cup almond flour

Directions:

1. Spray a 6- inch cake pan with cooking spray and set aside.
2. In a large bowl, mix together the almond flour, cinnamon, baking powder, swerve, and shredded coconut.
3. Add eggs, heavy cream, and coconut oil into the almond flour mixture and mix until well combined.
4. Pour batter into the prepared cake pan and cover the pan with foil.

5. Add 2 cups of water into the instant pot, then place a steamer rack in the pot.
6. Place cake pan on top of steamer rack.
7. Seal the instant pot with the lid and select manual high pressure and set the timer for 40 minutes.
8. Once the timer goes off, allow to release pressure naturally for 10 minutes and then release using Quick-release method.
9. Open the lid carefully. Remove the cake pan from the pot and let it cool for 20 minutes.
10. Cut cake into slices and serve.

Nutrition:
- Calories: 228
- Fat: 21.7 g
- Carbohydrates: 5.2 g
- Protein: 5 g

Lemon Cheesecake

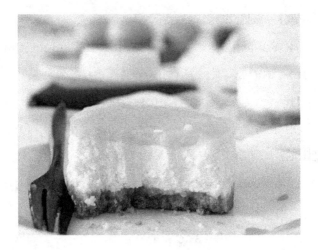

Preparation Time: 10 minutes

Cooking time: 35 minutes

Servings: 8

Ingredients:

For crust:

- 2 tablespoons coconut oil, melted
- 2 tablespoons swerve
- ¾ cup almond flour
- Pinch of salt

For filling:

- 2 tablespoons heavy whipping cream
- 2 large eggs

- 1 teaspoon lemon extract
- 1 teaspoon lemon zest
- 4 tablespoons fresh lemon juice
- 2/3 cup Swerve
- 1 lb cream cheese, softened

Directions:

1. Grease a 7-inch spring-form pan with butter and line with parchment paper. Set aside.
2. In a bowl, combine together all the crust ingredients and pour into the prepared pan and spread evenly, and place in the refrigerator for 15 minutes.
3. In a large mixing bowl, beat cream cheese using a hand mixer until smooth.
4. Add swerve, lemon extract, lemon zest, and lemon juice and beat again until just combined.
5. Add eggs and heavy whipping cream and beat until well combined.
6. Pour the filling mixture over the crust and spread evenly. Cover the springform pan with foil.
7. Pour 1 cup of water into the instant pot, then place a trivet in the pot.
8. Place cake pan on top of the trivet.
9. Seal instant pot with the lid and select manual high pressure for 35 minutes.

10. Allow releasing pressure naturally, then open the lid.

11. Remove the cake pan from the pot and let it cool completely.

12. Place in refrigerator for 3-4 hours.

13. Serve chilled and enjoy.

Nutrition:

- Calories: 322

- Fat: 31.1 g

- Carbohydrates: 4.4 g

- Protein: 8.3 g

Tasty Chocolate Cake

Preparation Time: 10 minutes

Cooking time: 30 minutes

Servings: 6

Ingredients:

- 3 large eggs
- ¼ cup butter, melted
- 1/3 cup heavy cream
- 1 teaspoon baking powder
- ¼ cup walnuts, chopped
- ¼ cup unsweetened cocoa powder
- 2/3 cup Swerve
- 1 cup almond flour

Directions:

1. Spray cake pan with cooking spray and set aside.
2. Add all ingredients into a large mixing bowl and mix using a hand mixer until the mixture looks fluffy.
3. Pour batter into the prepared cake pan.
4. Pour 2 cups of water into the instant pot, then place a steamer rack in the pot.
5. Place cake pan on top of steamer rack.

6. Seal the instant pot with the lid and cook on manual high pressure for 20 minutes.

7. Allow releasing pressure naturally for 10 minutes, then release using the Quick release method.

8. Open the lid carefully. Remove the cake pan from the pot and let it cool for 20 minutes.

9. Cut cake into slices and serve.

Nutrition:

- Calories: 275
- Fat: 25.5 g
- Carbohydrates: 7.5 g

Almond Spice Cake

Preparation Time: 10 minutes

Cooking time: 55 minutes

Servings: 10

Ingredients:

- 2 large eggs
- 2 cups almond flour
- 3 tablespoons walnuts (or pistachios), chopped
- ½ teaspoon vanilla
- 1/3 cup water
- 1/3 cup coconut oil, melted
- ¼ teaspoon ground cloves
- 1 teaspoon ground ginger
- 1 teaspoon cinnamon
- 2 teaspoon baking powder
- ½ cup Swerve
- Pinch of salt

Directions:

1. Spray a 7-inch cake pan with cooking spray and set aside.
2. Pour 1 cup of water into the instant pot, then place a trivet in the pot.

3. In a mixing bowl, whisk together the almond flour, cloves, ginger, cinnamon, baking powder, salt and swerve.

4. Stir in the eggs, vanilla, water, and coconut oil until combined.

5. Pour batter into the prepared cake pan and sprinkle chopped walnuts (or pistachios) on top. Cover the cake pan with foil and place it on top of the trivet in the instant pot.

6. Seal pot with lid and cook on manual high pressure for 40 minutes.

7. Allow releasing pressure naturally for 15 minutes. Open the lid carefully.

8. Remove the cake pan from the pot and let it cool for 20 minutes.

9. Cut cake into slices and serve.

Nutrition:

- Calories: 223
- Fat: 20.9 g
- Carbohydrates: 6.1 g
- Protein: 6.7 g

Walnut Carrot Cake

Preparation Time: 10 minutes

Cooking time: 50 minutes

Servings: 8

Ingredients:

- 3 large eggs
- ½ cup walnuts, chopped
- 1 cup carrots, shredded
- ½ cup heavy cream
- ¼ cup butter, melted
- 1 ½ teaspoon apple pie spice
- 1 teaspoon baking powder
- 2/3 cup Swerve
- 1 cup almond flour

Directions:

1. Spray a 6-inch cake pan with cooking spray and set aside.
2. Add all ingredients into the large mixing bowl and mix using a hand mixer until the mixture is well combined and looks fluffy.
3. Pour batter into the prepared cake pan and cover the pan with foil.

4. Pour 2 cups of water into the instant pot, then place a trivet in the pot.
5. Place cake pan on top of the trivet.
6. Seal pot with lid and cook on manual high pressure for 40 minutes.
7. Allow releasing pressure naturally for 10 minutes, then release using the Quick release method.
8. Open the lid carefully. Remove the cake pan from the pot and let it cool for 20 minutes.
9. Slice and serve.

Nutrition:

- Calories: 240

- Fat 22 g

- Carbohydrates: 6.2 g

- Protein: 7.6 g

Almond Cheesecake

Preparation Time: 10 minutes

Cooking time: 12 minutes

Servings: 6

Ingredients:

For crust:

- 3/4 cup almond flour
- 1 teaspoon swerve
- 2 tablespoons butter, melted

FOR CAKE:

- 2 eggs
- 1/4 cup sour cream
- 1 teaspoon vanilla
- 1/4 teaspoon liquid stevia
- 8 oz cream cheese, softened

Directions:

1. Grease a 7-inch spring-form pan with butter and line with parchment paper.
2. In a bowl, combine together almond flour, butter, and swerve. Transfer the crust mixture into the prepared pan and spread evenly.

3. In another bowl, beat together the liquid stevia and cream cheese until smooth.

4. Add egg one at a time. Add the sour cream and vanilla and beat until smooth.

5. Pour the cheese mixture on top of the crust and spread evenly. Cover the dish with foil.

6. Pour 2 cups of water into the instant pot and place trivet in the pot.

7. Place baking pan on top of the trivet.

8. Seal the instant pot with the lid and cook on manual high pressure for 12 minutes.

9. Allow releasing pressure naturally, then open the lid.

10. Remove the cake pan from the pot and let it cool completely.

11. Slice and serve.

Nutrition:

- Calories: 290
- Fat: 27.5 g
- Carbohydrates: 5 g
- Protein: 8 g

Vanilla Cheesecake

Preparation Time: 10 minutes

Cooking time: 30 minutes

Servings: 8

Ingredients:

- 8 oz cream cheese
- 2 eggs
- 1 teaspoon vanilla
- 2/3 cup Swerve
- 1 cup strawberries, sliced

Directions:

1. Grease a spring-form pan with butter and line with parchment paper. Set aside.
2. Add the cream cheese to a large bowl and beat using a hand mixer until smooth.
3. Add vanilla and swerve and blend until well combined.
4. Add eggs one at a time and blend until well combined.
5. Pour batter into the prepared pan. Cover pan tightly with foil.
6. Pour 1 cup of water into the instant pot, then place a trivet in the pot.

7. Place cake pan on top of the trivet.

8. Seal instant pot with the lid and select manual high pressure for 20 minutes.

9. Allow releasing pressure naturally for 10 minutes, then release using the quick release method.

10. Open the lid carefully. Remove the cake pan from the pot and let it cool completely.

11. Once the cake is completely cool, then arrange strawberry slices on top of the cake.

12. Cover cake with plastic wrap and place in refrigerator overnight.

13. Serve chilled and enjoy.

Nutrition:

- Calories: 122

- Fat: 11 g

- Carbohydrates: 2.5 g

- Protein: 3.6 g

Delicious Chocó Cheesecake

Preparation Time: 10 minutes

Cooking time: 15 minutes

Servings: 8

Ingredients:

- 2 eggs
- 2 teaspoons vanilla
- 1/4 cup sour cream
- 1/2 cup peanut flour
- 3/4 cup Swerve
- 16 oz cream cheese
- 1 tablespoon coconut oil
- 1/4 cup unsweetened chocolate chips
- 2 cups of water

Directions:

1. In a large bowl, beat cream cheese and swerve until smooth.
2. Gradually, add vanilla, sour cream, and peanut flour.
3. Add eggs one at a time and beat well to combine.
4. Spray a 4-inch spring-form pan with cooking spray.

5. Pour batter into the prepared pan and cover the pan with foil.
6. Pour 1 ½ cups of water into the instant pot, then place a trivet in the pot.
7. Place pan on top of the trivet.
8. Seal the instant pot with the lid and cook on manual high pressure for 15 minutes.
9. Allow releasing pressure naturally, then open the lid.
10. Remove the cake pan from the pot and let it cool completely.
11. In a microwave-safe bowl, add coconut oil and chocolate chips and microwave for 30 seconds. Stir well.
12. Drizzle melted chocolate over the cheesecake and place in the refrigerator for 1-2 hours.
13. Serve chilled and enjoy.

Nutrition:
- Calories: 315
- Fat: 28.9 g
- Carbohydrates: 5.3 g
- Protein: 8.2 g

Dark Chocolate Bars

Preparation Time: 10 minutes

Cooking time: 12 minutes

Servings: 4

Ingredients:

- 1 large egg
- 1 teaspoon stevia
- ½ cup unsweetened dark chocolate, grated
- 1 tablespoon unsweetened cocoa powder
- ½ cup almond butter
- ½ cup unsweetened almond milk
- 1 teaspoon vanilla
- 2 cups almond flour

Directions:

1. Pour 2 cups of water into the instant pot, then place a trivet in the pot.
2. Line a baking dish with parchment paper and set it aside.
3. Add all ingredients into the food processor and process until smooth.
4. Transfer mixture into the prepared baking dish and spread evenly with your hands.

5. Cover baking dish with foil and place on top of the trivet in the instant pot.

6. Seal the instant pot with the lid and select manual and set the timer for 12 minutes.

7. Release pressure using the quick-release method, then open the lid.

8. Remove the baking dish from the instant pot and let it cool for 20 minutes.

9. Cut the bar into slices and place in the refrigerator for 1-2 hours.

Nutrition:

- Calories: 321

- Fat: 26 g

- Carbohydrates: 13 g

CPSIA information can be obtained
at www.ICGtesting.com
Printed in the USA
LVHW061505190621
690652LV00003B/147

9 781802 697759